WAKE UP!

You're Alive, But

Are You Living?

40 simple self-care rituals for a healthy, abundant, and purposeful life

Allison Andrews

OmBody Health
Portland, ME

Dear Reader

This book represents the opinions and ideas of the author. The intention is to inspire you to reflect on behaviors, thought-patterns, beliefs, and habits that may be holding you back from achieving a healthier, more fulfilled existence. In no way does the author intend to undermine or fix your personal struggles.

The content of this book is for general instruction only. Each person's physical, emotional, and spiritual condition is unique. The instruction in this book is not intended to replace or interrupt your relationship with a physician or other professional. Please consult your doctor for matters pertaining to your specific health and diet.

This book is dedicated to my Nanny, who has never let me forget that I am exactly who I am meant to be and that I have a unique gift to offer the world. Nanny, your unwavering encouragement and support has helped me through the best and most challenging of times. You remind me to care for myself, slow down, and lighten up, and have never let me forget that I can do anything I put my mind to. Divine Order. I love you.

Contents

Acknowledgements

Belief in myself has not always come easy. Thank you to everyone who has ever believed in me, and reminded me to believe in myself: Mom and dad, Joe, my sisters, my grandparents, my clients, and the friends near and far who pull me up and offer me companionship when I need it most.

A special thanks to those who contributed their brains and creativity to this book. My editor, Emily Schweitzer, for your dedication, honest feedback, and encouragement. John and Sierra, thank you for your edits, guidance, and loving attention throughout this writing process. Leah Fisher Arsenault (cover photo and head shot) for your beautiful photos and creative vision.

I would not be the person I am today without my many spiritual and academic teachers: Wheaton professors, Indian Gurus, yoga teachers, Integrative Nutrition lecturers, inspirational authors. I thank you all for guiding me along my path toward health, personal development, and self-realization.

Lastly, my gratitude and affection goes out to all of my readers and clients for finding value in the wisdom that I have been so blessed to acquire in my life.

With love and appreciation, Allie

Foreword

For years, I struggled to maintain health and balance in my life. I would experience it here and there, and sense it deep down, but failed to sustain a consistent flow of regenerative lifestyle practices. While I strive to be a catalyst for positive and bold change in the world, my capacity to do so was undermined by a fundamental disconnect between my awareness and my actions. Thin-skinned, my core was shaken by the plight of others—and the planet.

To cope, I fell back on unhealthy habits like over consumption and began sacrificing my personal commitments for others. Feelings of shame and fatigue left me feeling crummy about myself all over again, perpetuating a negative feedback loop that did not align with my core values.

Working with Allie as a friend, coach and mentor has taught me to recognize old patterns as they arise and reinvest my energy in daily self-care practices. Through reciting daily affirmations and practicing the self-care techniques laid out in this book at my own pace, I am now able to rebound to a state of balance much quicker. Today, I feel more grounded in my body, my mind and my values. As Allie has illustrated through the wisdom laid out in this book, we cannot heal the wounds of the world until we first heal the wounds within ourselves. We can and must replenish natural and human systems and resources. It has become a moral obligation, and it starts with our personal stories.

It also starts with our choices.

To change self-limiting beliefs, I had to change my actions, and as I did, my beliefs transformed. All of a sudden, old story lines, impulse cravings, fear and judgments became obsolete. I didn't realize how much I had to gain until I created space for my own health to blossom. It was the courage to be honest with myself about who I am—and the life I aspire to lead—that opened the door for the life I now live. I feel like I am finally living in alignment with my life's purpose and path. As Allie conveys in each practice and affirmation, the propensity for awakening to our life's purpose exists within each one of us.

The key to activating abundant health lies in each moment through breath, clarity, and conviction.

This self-care guide offers a step-by-step path to follow in order to show up for your life each day with natural energy. The simple and advanced practices enclosed will support you in building a strong foundation to help you achieve optimal health and reach your goals. Practical tools and exercises will help you sharpen your ability to detect imbalance and overcome self-sabotage, shift your relationship with food, and take control of your personal stories. With courage and honesty, Allie Andrews weaves together a tapestry of accessible insights that can exist together, or independently—that meet you wherever you are and accelerate positive feedback loops within yourself and the world.

Sierra Flanigan
Director of Campus Sustainability &
Social Innovation at EcoMotion, Inc

"Integrity is wholeness...
The wholeness of life and things.
The divine beauty of the universe.
Love that, not man apart from that."
-Robinson Jeffers

Introduction

"It's not what we do once in a while that shapes our lives. It's what we do consistently."
-Anthony Robbins

I am so excited to share with you the tools that support my health, integrity, inner fulfillment, and sense of purpose. This book is written with firm self-awareness and an underlying belief that I control my destiny. The sense of control, self-awareness, and vitality that I feel has not always been so inherent. It took—and continues to take—daily practice to remain in this grounded place.

My hope is that this book guides you to feel more in control of your health and more alive. With daily practice we create a positive feedback loop in which our behaviors fuel our health and our health fuels our behaviors. We spiral into control.

Throughout the past few years, I have transformed into my healthiest self in mind and body. While I have always valued health, my actions did not consistently align with this value. Prior to my transformation, my confidence was low and sense of purpose nil. Most of the time, I was asleep for my life, anticipating the next distraction while disconnected from my true self and purpose.

At times I would eat healthfully, at times I would deprive myself, and at times I would turn to unhealthy foods and behaviors for satisfaction and distraction. My well-being was not consistent. Upon reflection, I realize that there was an underlying dissatisfaction; a void that I was masking with instant gratification, only to leave me feeling more dissatisfied later on. I did not feel in control. I was not awake to what brought me sustained enjoyment and fulfillment. I was not even close to living my fullest potential.

Now, I am someone who has made a decision to value and take care of my health every single day for the rest of my life. After significant reflection about what triggered this shift, I realized that the daily self-care practices described herein allowed me the space and time to investigate my dissatisfaction, change my mind, cultivate belief in myself, and be proactive.

I know that when I am not doing something in favor of my health every day—whether meditation, intentional breathing, eating a healthy meal, spending time with people who bring me up, fueling my passion, counting my blessings—I am less in control of my reality, and thus my destiny.

This book is not about my journey, but about the rituals that have supported me, and will continue to support me, in identifying and achieving my definition of success and optimal health.

The self-care practices described in this book are not my own, but a conglomerate of traditions and teachings that I have been blessed to acquire in my life. They are here to guide you toward achieving and maintaining *your* version of success and optimal health. When practiced persistently, the simple tools in this book can provide a nourishing foundation for total health and inner peace in a culture that values external gains and tells us that we must always be seeking more.

What is Self-Care?

Self-care is an expression of self-love. It encompasses any deliberate action taken by an individual to uphold and enhance their health and well being. My experiences and education have taught me that health is individual—what supports my health, may be different than what supports yours—and multidimensional—it needs to be nurtured on multiple levels. Thus, self-care is not only about taking care of our bodies, but on a deeper level it is getting to know ourselves—tuning into and making time for the behaviors, activities, rituals, foods, environments, people, thoughts, and beliefs that support our health and personal development. The self-care practices in this book work on both the body and the mind.

The Wisdom of Yoga

Yoga is to gain mastery over the mind.
-Patanjali, Yoga Sutras (400 CE)

Much of the insight provided in this book stems from the wisdom of yoga, an Indian tradition dating back at least 5,000 years. Today, there are many definitions, branches, and translations of this ancient tradition, including the definition above. However, the underlying paradigm remains: yoga is self-realization. The yogic tradition provides us with a path along which we can fulfill our potential and get more enjoyment out of life. Along the way, we adopt practices that help us remain gracious, present, and focused in our day-to-day life. Although often misunderstood as a series of physical postures, yoga is a lifestyle that supports and unites the whole person (mind, body, soul and spirit).

I have been acquiring this yogic wisdom for over eleven years and the most important lesson I've learned is that regular practice pays off. It wasn't until I started practicing consistently—not just asana (posture), but pranayama (controlling the flow of vital life force energy with the breath), meditation, shatkarma (cleansing practices for the body)—that the concept of yoga as a lifestyle started to make sense to me.

Overtime, I transformed from someone who was lacking confidence and easily ruffled, into someone who is secure, resilient, patient, calm, and present for my life. I finally felt what the ancient yogic text, *The Yoga Sutras* by Patanjali, tries to communicate: *Sthira Sukham Asanam (steadiness, ease, presence of mind)*—a sense of strength and control, with an underlying lightness, effortlessness, and the ability to let go.

I share all of this to communicate the importance of staying true to your practice and true to yourself—once you figure out what works for you, stick with it. Notice what arises when you waiver, and then get right back to your practice.

> *"Yoga is 99% practice and 1% theory."*
> —Sri K. Pattabhi Jois

The powerful reality of this statement cannot be realized until experienced. And the transformative benefits of ritualistic self-care cannot be appreciated or fulfilled until the practices are integrated with diligence and awareness. Daily practice is the key to lasting transformation and self-realization.

How to Use This Book

I have tried to make this book as simple, short, and to the point as possible. I want you to stop reading about self-care and start doing it, today. Adopt these rituals slowly, methodically, and with great awareness for what you are experiencing in mind and body as you integrate them into your day.

The sequence of rituals is fitting: the practices toward the beginning are simple and designed to lay a foundation for those that follow. For someone who is already taking intentional action in favor of their health daily, feel free to jump around and pick the activities that resonate with you. As you perform these rituals, observe your sensory experiences, your breath, and your thoughts. Be aware of any resistance that arises, both as you read and as you practice. In the beginning, shifting your thoughts and behaviors will likely feel forced, but in time the fruits of your diligence will begin to radiate throughout your entire being.

I cannot tell you how to nurture yourself in order to realize your potential, but I can offer you a list of daily practices that can bring you closer to identifying what you need to do to be your best self. I hope the sequence of practices herein guide you toward discovering what you are capable of.

Affirmations

Each chapter starts with an affirmation. An affirmations is an assertive, present-tense statement of something as fact.

9

Usually spoken as *I am* or *I have* statements, affirmations are powerful tools to shift your thinking, cultivate belief in yourself, and create the present and the future that you want.

Affirmations are a self-care practice in and of themselves. They can be whispered silently, each day, maybe on repeat. At first, you may not believe the affirmation, and this is a completely normal reaction of the ego (one dimension of the self that can hold significant power and have skewed perceptions of reality). But as you repeat the affirmation, visualize the outcome, and remain present for what arises, eventually the affirmation will begin to sound more like truth (for guidance see Self-Awareness Exercise 1, page 16). You will move from incredulity to wavering belief, from wavering belief to commitment, from commitment to certainty, and before you know it, that which you have affirmed has been manifested.

*   *   *   *   *

Health does not have to feel ascetic. Taking care of our minds and bodies does not have to feel like a burden, we do not have to feel deprived. Once we start cultivating positivity and health through daily practice, we have less time for thoughts, behaviors, and foods that do not support our well-being and success. And then something truly remarkable starts happening; when viewing the word through a lens of health and self-awareness, we are more satisfied with our life and no longer feel the need to distract ourselves with behaviors and foods that deplete our well being. Our taste buds wake up and nutritious food tastes better than junk food. Health-promoting behaviors become an integral part of our daily life. We are resilient; when we get off track, we are aware and jump right back on with a sense of eager acceptance and ease. We are less distracted by lethargy, brain fog, angst, perceived failures, and self-sabotage. We are more present for our life and those in it. We wake up and feel more alive.

Before journeying into the specific self-care practices laid out in this book, Chapter One will guide you through developing awareness for thought patterns and beliefs that are holding you back. We have to identify and work through the barriers to change before transformation is possible.

Chapter One

Affirm Your Abundance and Success

Affirmation
I have everything I need within; anything external only augments my happiness.

Do you ever get lost in the dream of not having or being enough? I refer to this way of thinking as a scarcity mindset: perceptions of what we lack, often infused with negative judgments or blame of ourselves, others, and circumstances. A scarcity mindset often prevents us from taking full responsibility for areas in our life where we are dissatisfied; thus, can hold us back from taking initiative to turn our dreams and affirmations into reality.

I used to live my life from a place of scarcity. Rather than noticing all that was plentiful in my life, my awareness tended toward what was wrong, what was lacking: *I don't have enough time, I don't know enough, I'm too skinny, I'm too fat, I'm not making enough money, I'm not smart enough, I could never do that, I'll never find true love, I'm not confident.*

These are examples of limiting beliefs: the stories we identify with that instill fear and hold us back from taking action; thus, creating more scarcity and discontent in our lives. Because they are the result of a lifetime of meaningful experiences, interactions, and upbringings, limiting beliefs are often deeply engrained and feel like part of us. However, with practice and awareness this tendency toward self-defeating thought patterns can be squashed.

In order to train ourselves out of a scarcity mindset, we must nurture an outlook of abundance: awareness and appreciation for the plentitude of beauty and good in our daily lives with the courage to take action. In order to nurture an abundance mindset, we must be pro-active in noticing what is going well everyday, no matter how obvious: *I am alive, I'm breathing, I am loved, I love, I have the capacity to help others, the sun is shining, I have work, I have money, I have time, I can* [fill in the blank].

Unlike the scarcity mindset which limits action, the abundance mindset inspires action; thus, manifesting as self-control, plenitude, and success in our lives. In the abundance frame of thinking, we are aware of and take one hundred percent responsibility for dissatisfaction in a given area of our life. We do not wallow in a state of blame or self-pity; rather, we recognize that it is up to us to take action to address discontent by making a tangible change or shifting our thinking.

A Note to Busy People

Busy people make things happen.

You're busy. You may have kids, a sick parent, an all-

14

encompassing job, or something else that sucks up your time. I do not mean to imply that feeling busy is the same as existing in a scarcity mindset. You likely feel crunched for time on a daily basis, but when you approach this feeling from a place of self-awareness, accountability and abundance, you can recognize when you start to fall into limiting, scarcity-ridden thought patterns. What does this scarcity mindset do to your energy and productivity?

For example: There is a difference between the thought process, *I have 10-minutes to get this done, I better get moving!* And, *I don't have enough time.* The first is an abundance-oriented thought because it recognizes the time you *do* have. While the second is limiting, leaving a residue of fear, anxiety and stress because it is based on the assumption of not having enough or getting enough done.

Being busy is not a bad thing. You have immense opportunity every day to create and re-create your life and identity by shifting your beliefs to reflect a positive, abundance-oriented outlook.

Tip: Carve out time in your busy day to be intentional and practice self-care by setting reminders on your phone.

* * * * *

External abundance comes and goes, but the outlook of abundance can stay with you forever. By putting a little time into the self-care practices that follow, you can evolve an abundance mindset. In time, you can and will wake up each day with the underlying belief that you have everything you need, that everything is okay, more than okay, that you are spectacular.

Of course, you will still experience bouts of doubt,

fear, sadness, scarcity, dis-ease and pain, but—so long as you are practicing daily care—such perceptions and feelings will come to you more lightly and less often, with an inner knowing that all is well. Like a flame, this inner knowing must be tended to. The more we tend to it, the brighter it burns and the more in control we feel of our destiny. The less we tend to it, the more it flickers and the more we get lost in the dream of scarcity. (Hence the need for daily practice.)

Developing Self-Awareness

In order to shift your thinking, it is first important to develop awareness around your current tendencies and limiting beliefs. Sometimes these self-defeating thoughts are so deeply engrained within our psychology that we cannot even recognize them. For example, have you ever looked at something someone else has done and thought: *I could never do that?* Given how deeply engrained many of our critical thought patterns are, they can be difficult to notice and therefore let go of.

How do we change a self-defeating belief system? We approach these fear-based thoughts head on. Rather than ignoring them, we choose to be fully present for fear and doubt within our self. While this is likely to cause immediate discomfort, by approaching rather than ignoring these self-defeating thoughts, we intentionally create space for the belief, the positivity, that we can, that we will.

It takes time to build certainty in ourselves after so many years of being told (by our own mind or others) that we cannot, but with consistent practice, thought awareness, and affirmation, we can truly change the mind.

16

By simply initiating the process of creating space for the idea that we can set and achieve the goals we desire, a world of opportunity opens up that we never would have approached.

Soon you will begin to create space for the belief that you can and will do whatever you set your mind to. It is from this belief, this thought, that you transform from someone who is inhibited by their sense of scarcity within reality, into someone who consciously creates a reality of abundance and purpose.

Thoughts are powerful.

"Whatever you think, that you will be. If you think yourself weak, weak you will be; if you think yourself strong, strong you will be."
–Swami Vivekananda

What we believe creates who we are. What we believe about ourselves creates our identity. It takes great awareness to recognize and shift our beliefs—especially about ourselves—because they are often so deeply engrained in our psyche. What are your limiting beliefs? Is there something you want to do or feel, but your beliefs are holding you back?

In order to shed some light on the beliefs that may be limiting your potential, we are going to do this thought experiment. Use Self-Awareness Exercise 1 on page 16 to shed light on one or more of your limiting beliefs. Come up with an affirmation (an *I*, *I am*, or *I have* statement) that will guide you toward shifting this scarcity belief to create space for positive thought, self-awareness, and personal development.

*   *   *   *   *

Belief in yourself is like a seed, a kernel of potential; without it, you cannot grow, but its presence alone does not necessarily mean that you will triumph. In order for that seed to grow to its fullest, it needs a nourishing foundation. Thus, an important component of affirming our success and abundance is building and maintaining a foundation of health. A foundation that is not reinforced or damaged by accomplishments and perceived failures, but that is maintained by daily self-care and self-love.

With daily self-care and affirmation we encourage body-mind awareness, healthy behaviors, and positive psychology, all of which support our success and abundance. Furthermore, the path to daily care outlined in the chapters that follow support the outlook that success and abundance are not dependent on our continually changing external world. Our joy exists now and always, we just have to take the time to tune in and nurture it.

Self-Awareness Exercise 1

Write down a limiting belief and affirmation. For example:

Belief: *I want to meditate every day, but I don't have enough time.*

Or

I am an awful public speaker; I get so nervous.

Affirmation: *I meditate for 10-minutes every day.*

Or

I am an inspirational public speaker; I exude confidence.

Now, close your eyes and repeat your affirmation to yourself. Notice what thoughts come up surrounding your affirmation. Is there discomfort or an underlying disbelief that you will never get there? What excuses, stories or past experiences arise? For example:

I will never make the time to meditate everyday. I never follow through with anything I do. What's the point of doing it today, I know I won't do it tomorrow.

Or

I don't have the confidence to speak in front of others. I don't have anything special to offer. I don't know enough, why would anyone listen to me?

Be present for what arises. Do not push your fears or doubts away, experience them. Decide to take the next opportunity to be proactive in shifting your limiting belief. For example:

I will wake up 10-minutes earlier tomorrow and meditate.

Or

I will take the next opportunity to lead by example, speak my mind, and teach what I know.

Do this exercise every single day until you truly believe your affirmation. Write your affirmation down and put it somewhere obvious. Soon, your actions will reflect what you wish for yourself, but you must take action (see page 130).

Notes

Limiting Beliefs:

Affirmations:

Notes

What arises as you state your affirmations?

Note: If you are having trouble believing your affirmations, your can state them in a way that feels more approachable, more real. For example: *"I am working on meditating every day."* or *"I am in the process of becoming a public speaker."*

Chapter Two

Make a Habit of Self-Care and Self-Love

Affirmation
I choose self-love, health and vitality.

Self-love and compassion are fundamental to optimal health. You may have noticed that when you have loving thoughts, you are less likely to distract yourself from feelings of contempt with toxic (self-sabotaging) behaviors, such as over-eating foods that take away from your health and vitality. Loyally caring for your body is an excellent way to soften your relationship with yourself, reduce toxic thoughts and behaviors, and build a nourishing foundation off of which you can blossom.

> *"To keep the body in good health is a duty... otherwise we shall not be able to keep our mind strong and clear."*
> —Buddha

Many of the practices that follow are designed to eliminate toxins from the body. Toxins are poisonous substances that can build up in the body either via ingestion, absorption through the skin, or as natural bi-products of cellular metabolism and energy production (increased when we eat the Standard American Diet—see Chapter Four, page 85).

The liver, kidneys, and lungs work hard to cleanse the body of toxic waste products every single day, but when the daily burden is great—due to exposure to environmental pollutants, poor diet, low functioning detox organs, and even toxic thinking (scarcity mindset and negative thought patterns)—the system can get overwhelmed leading to poor health. Poor health is a sign of systemic imbalance, affecting multiple organ systems, cellular and energetic processes in the body, and our thinking.

Chapter One works on your thinking because the nature of your thoughts determines your behaviors and visa versa; thus, physical health and mental health are innately intertwined. Poor health correlates with heaviness in body—extra weight, stale energy, and a heavy toxic burden—which often reflects as heaviness in mind—unceasing, scarcity-driven thoughts, limiting beliefs, and a tendency to hold on tightly to the past. Whereas optimal health correlates with lightness in body and mind—little to no toxic buildup, little fat around the organs, a vibrant energy, and the ability to let go. (It is important to note, the "lightness in body" does not necessarily indicate a slim figure; some people are naturally heavier set at their healthiest, lightest state. Additionally, an individual may be slim but still exude heaviness due to toxic burden and/or visceral fat.)

As you reduce your body's toxic burden, you will begin to create space for a renewed sense of

24

being. For those who tend toward a scarcity mindset (as described in Chapter One), daily self-care can be effective in detoxifying your thinking and cleansing your outlook of limiting beliefs.

I do not think that we have to be extremists when it comes to our health, but it does help if we are acting in favor of our health every single day—for detoxification and otherwise. Use the practices in this chapter to ritualize caring for yourself and make a habit of prioritizing your health. Consider the following rituals a demonstration of self-love and self-respect and make an effort to cultivate loving, abundance–oriented thoughts as you practice. Remain accountable to yourself by doing at least one of these rituals every single day this week.

"Every choice we make can be a celebration of the world [and life] we want."
-Frances Moore Lappe

-1-

Clean Your Tongue

*An indispensible practice in some parts of the world,
this practice removes toxins, maintains oral hygiene,
and boosts health- and self-awareness.*

Have you ever noticed a white filmy coating on your tongue when you wake up in the morning? As we sleep, we enter into a restorative, healing state where our bodies work to "clean up" or detoxify. Some of these excreted toxins work their way up the digestive tract and get deposited on the tongue. Cleaning your tongue removes excreted toxins, preventing their reabsorption into the body, and reducing your body's overall toxic burden.

When: Avoid re-ingestion of toxins by making this the first thing you do in the morning, before drinking water.

How Often: Everyday

The Practice: Use a metal spoon or purchase a tongue-cleaning device at your local health food store or online. An ideal tongue cleaner is a curved apparatus made of copper, tin, brass, silver, gold or stainless steel with soft edges. Scrape from the back forward 8 to 15 times without using too much pressure (this shouldn't hurt or cause bleeding), rinsing the tongue scraper with water every 3 to 4 scrapes.

Benefits: Combats bad breath; improves oral hygiene; detoxifies the mouth and digestive tract; reduces overall toxic burden on the body; enhances taste sensitivity; reduces cravings; boosts immunity.

-2-

Drink Lots of Water in the Morning

An essential daily practice for better digestion, nutrient absorption, and brain function.

We are fluid beings. Your body is 70% water and that water needs to be continually replenished. When we sleep, our cellular processes and bodily functions remain active (although slower); thus, we become dehydrated. Drinking water in the morning is a simple, yet integral part of your daily self-care routine.

When: In the morning, after cleaning your tongue and at least 20 minutes before eating or drinking coffee.

The Practice: It's simple, pour yourself 20 to 30 ounces (up to 2 liters if you can tolerate it) of room temperature water and drink as you go about your morning routine. If 20 ounces seems like a lot, start with just a small glass of water and increase a little each day or week.

Benefits: Boosts metabolism; hydrates and replenishes your cells; increases the production of new blood and muscle cells; purges the blood of toxins for clear skin; feeds the brain (which is 75-85% water); stimulates intestinal peristalsis (wave-like contractions in the gastrointestinal tract) to support digestion; purifies the colon to support the absorption of nutrients.

Oil Pulling

An ancient cleansing practice for the mouth said to bring balance to the entire body. At the very least, this practice will improve your oral hygiene and whiten your teeth!

When: In the morning, on an empty stomach, after cleaning your mouth. Ideally, this practice is done an hour after drinking water or tea.

How Often: Can be practiced daily to maintain balance in your body, but is especially effective in cases of acute and chronic illness. If you are sick, you can practice oil pulling on an empty stomach 3 times per day to remove toxins (before meals).

The Practice: Use sesame oil, coconut oil or sunflower oil. Put about 2 tablespoons of oil into your mouth and swish around for 20 minutes. Set a timer so you don't exceed this amount of time. As the oil starts to pick up toxins, it becomes white, frothy and thick. It is at this point that you should spit it out into the trash or outside (not in the sink) before the toxins are reabsorbed into your mouth. Rinse your mouth a few times with warm water.

Tip: Depending on how much time you have, this practice can be done while sitting quietly, showering, stretching, or planning for the day.

Benefits: Cleanses the mouth and body; whitens the teeth; reduces toxic load for more energy and clearer skin; improves oral hygiene for better overall health; brings the body into greater balance by cleansing the mouth of toxins.

-4-

Neti Pot

*A refreshing practice to clean the nasal passage and a
natural remedy for ear, nose, and throat conditions.
This practice is both therapeutic and preventative.*

IMPORTANT! This practice must be paired with Practice 14: Skull Shining Breath (page 62). Post-neti pot, do as many rounds of Skull Shining Breath as needed to get all of the water out of your nose; this is important to prevent cold or flu. For instruction, see pages 62 – 64. After Kapalbhati, you may put a drop of organic sesame or olive oil in the nose to prevent it from drying out.

When: In the morning, before eating, or anytime throughout the day. Avoid preforming on a full stomach.

How Often: As often as everyday to promote youth and good health. This practice is especially beneficial if you're experiencing ear, nose, and throat infection, excess mucus, congestion, and/or energy imbalance (overtired or over-stimulated).

The Practice: A neti pot can be purchased at your local health food store or online. A ceramic pot will be best for long-term use. In your neti pot, dissolve ¼ teaspoon organic, non-iodized salt per 8 oz of warm, clean water. Practice over the tub, sink or outdoors. Lean foreword and tilt your head to the right, placing the neti pot spout in the left nostril. Tilt the pot and let the salted water drain out through the opposite (right) nostril. Breathe through your mouth. Drain ½ to 1 full neti pot (depending on severity of congestion) and repeat on the opposite side.

Tip: If you're experiencing any burning sensation in the nose, you don't have the correct water to salt ratio (you added too much or too little salt).

Benefits: Improves breathing, taste, and smell; removes mucus and relieves sinus problems; balances energy channels in the body.

33

Sesame Oil Massage

Self massage will relax and soothe your muscles, while stimulating blood flow and moisturizing to keep the skin smooth and supple.

When: Fifteen minutes before showering or just after you have showered (experiment with both and see which works best for you).

How Often: As often as you would like. Every time you shower for optimal results.

The Practice: Simply massage yourself from head-to-toe with oil, paying special attention to any areas with tension or pain (such as the shoulders, neck or, quads after an intense workout). And don't forget the bottoms of the feet and between the toes!

Tip: Oil can also be applied while in the sauna. Putting the legs up against the wall and massaging the legs with oil will stimulate blood flow from the lower extremities and support detoxification. You can even nourish your scalp by oil massaging once a week (before your shower). Coconut oil can also be used.

Benefits: A natural anti-bacterial for wounds or infections; reduces inflammation; reduces premature aging; moisturizes the skin; can be a treatment for eczema, dry, or itchy skin; restores hair's natural balance and luster; stimulates the release of toxins in the body; relaxes and calms the body and mind.

-6-

Hot Towel Scrub

This loving practice is calming, exfoliating, detoxifying, and a great way to pay tribute to your body.

When: In the evenings, before bed, or anytime you're feeling in need of some calm and self-love.

How Often: I'll let you decide.

The Practice: Fill your bathroom sink with warm water. Use a warm washcloth to scrub your skin. Be intentional, start with the face and chest, then move to each arm (develop your own process). Spend extra time massaging the lymph nodes under the armpits and in the groin area to stimulate the lymphatic system.

Tip: It may be tempting to do this practice in the shower, but it is more effective and intentional when done standing by the sink. Make this a scared part of your day, just for you, by lighting a candle or using essential oils.

Benefits: Exfoliates the skin; reduces muscle tension; energizes in the morning; relaxes in the evening; opens pores and releases toxins; activates circulatory and lymphatic systems; reflects self-love.

-7-

Honey Mask

A natural way to promote smooth, clean, and radiant skin.

When: I usually do this practice in the evenings, after a long day, or in the morning for glowing skin.

How Often: As often as you'd like for optimal benefits.

The Practice: Wash or rinse your face. Massage raw organic honey into your skin. Leave the honey on your face for anywhere from 10 to 30 minutes. Rinse honey off with warm water, no soap is needed.

Tip: After rinsing, splash cold water on your open eyes to exercise the eye muscles.

Benefits: Honey's natural antibacterial, antiseptic, and antioxidant properties make its benefits far reaching: Cleans the skin; treats acne, pimples, infections, wounds, and scars; prevents premature aging; reduces skin damage.

Hot Water Bottle

This self-soothing practice is both comforting and pain-relieving after a long day.

When: During sleep, to relax, or to ease cramps or digestive discomfort.

How Often: Can be used each night, especially during the winter.

The Practice: Purchase a soft, rubber hot water bottle from your local pharmacy or simply use a hard plastic bottle (such as a Nalgene). Fill your vessel with hot water. If the water is boiling, be sure to wrap the bottle with a towel so you don't burn yourself.

Tips: Place the hot water bottle on your feet for warmth, on your back for strain, on the lower abdomen for cramps, and on the abdomen to stimulate digestion (after a big meal).

I like to place a hot water bottle on my belly, close my eyes and practice Soft Belly Breathing (see Practice 11, page 56 and 57) as I fall asleep at night.

Benefits: Relaxes sore muscles and the entire body/mind; eases menstrual cramps; warms the bed; eases arthritic pain (especially in the hands); calming; provides comfort and warmth; weighted heat on the belly releases stored tension and trauma in the solar plexus area.

-9-

Drink Tulsi Tea

Tulsi, or holy basil, is an adaptogenic* herb revered in many Eastern traditions for its therapeutic and stress-beating capabilities.

*Adaptogens are powerful immune boosters that help the body deal with stress and toxins at a cellular level.

When: Morning, noon, and night (anytime). A great way to start and end the day, or an excellent mid-afternoon pick-me-up.

How Often: If you're someone who gets easily agitated, stressed, or has anxiety and/or insomnia, drink as many as two cups per day.

Tip: Drink extra Tulsi tea while traveling, moving, or going through challenging times to help the body cope with changing environments and stressors.

Benefits: Restores natural balance in the body; balances adrenal function and hormones; decreases sensitivity to stress and free radicals (toxins) on a cellular level; helps the body cope with internal stressors like anxiety, insomnia and changing hormones.

Note: Nature provides us with many adaptogens, including: Chaga, Reishi (mushrooms), Ashwagandha, Chinese Ginseng, and Liccorice Root, many of which are available as tinctures, powders, or capsules. These herbal tonics are powerful, so be sure to research the benefits and contra-indications prior to use.

*   *   *   *   *

As you make self-care a habit, pay extra attention to what you are feeling. I can tell you that something will benefit you, but if it does not feel good, you may choose to re-evaluate. As a society, we tend to over-value thinking and under-value feeling. Just as thoughts are information, what we feel provides equally valuable information to drive our decisions and actions. Additionally, both thoughts and feelings can be misconstrued, leading to a lack of clarity and triggering us to behave in ways that spiral us out of control. For example: binging on food or alcohol, saying things that we do not mean, or becoming consumed in negative thinking about ourselves, others, or our circumstances.

The remaining practices provide tools to peel away the layers that often lead to misinterpretation or unawareness of thoughts and feelings, such as heaviness in mind and body, lethargy, stress, and fear. From here we move forward to strengthen the skill of self-awareness.

Chapter Three

Develop the Skill of Mindfulness

Affirmation
"Thank you so much, I am happy, I am healthy, I have no complaints whatsoever." –Dr. Bernie Seigal

As we have learned, our foundation of health needs constant reinforcement. The next step to achieving health and abundance is developing a more mindful and enlightened outlook.

According to the Buddhist tradition, enlightenment is the spiritual state of non-attachment to people, things, and outcomes. To many of us, enlightenment seems almost impossible to achieve in our culture where so much of what we are motivated by is external.

"If the earth needs night as well as day, wouldn't it follow that the soul requires endarkenment to balance enlightenment."
–Tom Robbins, Jitterbug Perfume

Even enlightened beings will succumb to "endarkenment"—attachment, judgment, and commitment to an outcome. However, we can use daily practice to cultivate a more mindful and enlightened outlook on our attachments, judgments, successes, and perceived failures.

So, what is mindfulness? As Angela Melzer (Minds in Motion, CO) put it so eloquently,

"To be mindful, is to kindly attend to your moment without judging it."

For the purposes of this book, "judgment" means the tendency to label an emotion, place, behavior, person, or the self favorably or unfavorably. Based on these definitions, an example of mindfulness would be: Being present for the anxiety you might feel before a job interview—or other occasion when you feel the need to "prove yourself". In this case, mindfulness means you remain aware of the temptation to get lost in limiting beliefs or expectations of what might happen, but instead of spiraling down this thought pattern of "what if", choosing to let go of outcomes and to shift your awareness back to the present, back to the breath (or repeat an affirmation—*I always do my best, I radiate confidence, I believe in myself.*)

But what about when we *do* judge? When we really start to investigate the word "judgment", we will see that we do it all the time. It is not only natural to judge our present moment, but a necessary component of decision-making. Initially, awareness of the nature of our judgments is more important than resisting the tendency to judge. For example, judgments can be self-defeating and bring us down—as in the outlook of scarcity—or ego-promoting and expectation forming—as when our happiness and self-worth depend heavily on our external world of relationships, accomplishments, jobs, and other things that tend to shape our self-esteem.

It is not a bad thing to bask in our achievements and external gains, or reflect on how we could have done something differently, but we must be aware when we put too much weight on these temporary components of existence. Once we find peace in the fact that if it all came crashing down we would still be ok (*I have everything I need within*), we will be able to find peace in any situation. From this perspective, we recognize that our joy and suffering are not contingent on the external world and its stimuli, and we intentionally remain present and appreciative for the richness of daily life.

*   *   *   *   *

The next fundamental piece of mindfulness is compassion. Compassion for when we do make harsh judgments, for when we do have resistance, and for when things are not going the way we hoped. Thus far we have been cultivating self-awareness, self-love, and self-respect with affirmations and practices that purge the body and mind of toxic residue. Now it is time to work on self-compassion, or softening to yourself (and finding acceptance when necessary) in light of self-defeating judgments or behaviors. With compassion comes the ability to let go of the past and move forward.

Self-compassion does not mean complacency. To be truly mindful is to consciously take ourselves out of the present moment when necessary in order to actively reflect on how we can advance ourselves and our thinking.

When we put it all together, mindfulness is the skill of compassionately observing our judgments, actions, and reactions; or more simply, mindfulness is compassionate self-awareness. In this day, age, and culture, compassionate awareness is the closest most of us will come to enlightenment. Coupled with self-love and self-respect, mindfulness is foundational to manifesting a mindset and life of abundance and purpose.

How Do We Develop the Skill of Mindfulness?

To create space in the mind for a more enlightened outlook, we must carve out time each day to practice being present and mindful. As we practice being present, we must recognize that it is in the very nature of the mind to have wandering and judgmental thoughts. Lost somewhere in the transition from childhood to adulthood, present moment awareness is a skill that needs to be nurtured and re-learned, over and over again.

The following breathing and meditation practices (also referred to as awareness practices) come from the yogic tradition and when practiced diligently can change the course of your entire life. Yoga will open up your body and mind, eliminating unnecessary stress, tension, and heaviness, healing your entire being, and supporting a mindful outlook.

Practice Tips

Although not addressed in this text, the benefits of the physical dimension of yoga—postures or asanas—are far-reaching and can undoubtedly support your health and self-awareness. If you do not already have an asana practice, I highly recommend seeking the guidance of an experienced teacher to develop this supportive element in your life. That said, a physical practice is not necessary to do yoga.

> *"As long as you can breathe, you can do yoga."*
> –Patanjali

Use the following tips to achieve maximum benefits and enjoyment from the awareness practices that succeed.

When to Practice: Generally, the best time to practice yoga is in the morning, when the belly is empty and the mind is clear; however, any practice is better than no practice!

When choosing a time for your daily awareness practice, it can be beneficial to pick a time of day when you feel the most distracted or out of control—such as when you feel stressed, tend to overeat, or spiral into a scarcity mindset. Alternatively, if you have children or other obligations, you should schedule your practice during a time when you can devote your full attention to yourself and your practice. Ideally, we perform these techniques on an empty stomach because when the stomach is full (of food or drink) it compresses the lungs causing distraction and discomfort.

Duration of Practice: Start by carving out just 5 minutes each day for Breath Control (see Practice 10, page 54 and 55). This helps to build a daily habit and ritual. After a couple of weeks, you can make a point to elevate your awareness practice, first working up to 10 and then 20 minutes per day, and eventually 20 minutes two times per day. As you get to this point, you can use any of the breathing techniques that follow to lead into and/or close your meditation practice (see page 65). However, keep in mind that Breath Control (Practice 10) can be effective in supporting a more mindful outlook in as little as one to three breaths.

Where to Practice: When first starting out, try to practice in a quiet place with minimal distraction. Practicing in a room by yourself with the door closed allows you to fully commit to your practice without the interruption of people or pets.

Cell Phone: Put your cell pone on airplane mode. This way, you can use it to keep the time, without getting distracted by text messages, emails, or calls. Download a Meditation Timer App so that you do not get sidetracked by checking the time.

Sitting Posture: For the following practices, choose a comfortable sitting position in which you can sit tall. It is important to lengthen your spine and maintain an open chest to create more space for the breath. For some, this may mean sitting cross-legged on the floor or on a cushion, but for most this means sitting in a chair with the back supported. In this case, allow your head to be free, resisting the urge to lean back, as this might result in you falling asleep. (If you do fall asleep, it is likely that you are sleep deprived. This is your body's way of telling you to get more sleep. If you have time, let yourself doze off. As you restore yourself via the rituals in this book, you will be able to enter into a deeply relaxed, restful state without falling asleep).

Awareness: Notice what comes up for you; sensations, thought patterns, stories? Try not to dwell on thoughts or search for something profound. Acknowledge your thoughts, and then let them go. Gently and with compassion bring yourself back to your breath or focal point. It is normal for your mind to wander, the mindful part of these practices is the ability to bring your attention back to the present.

Note: In the yoga tradition there are many variations of the breathing and meditation techniques that follow. For the purposes of this book, these practices are kept simple. To deepen and expand on any yoga practice, seek the guidance of an experienced teacher.

*   *   *   *   *

Be present for what arises as you create space physically, mentally, and spiritually for a new way of being. As you deepen your awareness practice, you will create the space necessary for letting go of or confronting something you have been grasping or avoiding. This process can feel challenging and uncomfortable, but is often necessary for personal growth and transformation. Throughout this process, have fun getting to know yourself. When in doubt, nurture self-compassion.

51

Breathing Practices

"Feelings come and go like clouds in a windy sky. Conscious breathing is my anchor."
—Thich Nhat Hanh

The breath is the most accessible path to the present moment. Intentional breathing is extremely effective for mitigating stress, calming the mind, balancing the nervous system, and generally bringing the body and mind into greater equilibrium.

On a cellular level, the breath is vital, energizing, and purifying. As we breathe deeply, we are flooding the blood with oxygen, essential for proper cellular functioning. Deep breathing is also effective in exercising the respiratory organs to maintain breath capacity, which is diminished as we age.

The following breathing techniques come from the yogic tradition called pranayama, which means controlling vital life force energy with breath. The techniques provided here are basic, yet when done properly and consistently, are extremely effective in balancing physical and subtle energies in the body. They are labeled beginner, intermediate, and advanced so that you can learn them in proper order and achieve the most benefit. Do not worry about getting them perfect in the beginning, just focus on doing them. With time and practice, they will become second nature.

Disclaimer: Please keep in mind that controlling the flow of life force energy into, within, and out of the body can have powerful psychophysical effects. If you're suffering from a condition such as high blood pressure, heart disease, neurological conditions or depression, and for those who are pregnant, it is recommended that you do further research before integrating the following breathing practices.

-10-

Breath Control

Beginner

This practice will allow present moment awareness to penetrate your daily life.

Breath control is an excellent tool anytime you feel the stress response kick in—heat, tension, nervousness, racing thoughts—because it mitigates fight-or-flight (see page 67) by reducing chronic cortisol and re-focusing the mind on the task at hand.

The Practice: Simply breathe in and out through your nose, softly, smoothly and as quiet or silent as you can. If breathing out through your nose is uncomfortable for you, or you're feeling overheated, let the breath out through your mouth. In time, you will be able to breathe in and out through the nose comfortably.

As you develop this skill, focus on controlling the length of the inhale to match the length of the exhale. Breathing in to a silent count of 4 to 6 seconds (or longer) and breathing out for the same count. Counting helps to maintain an even breath and provides a focal point for the mind. At first, you may feel the need to draw lots of air in quickly (you'll know you're doing this if your breath is loud); instead, focus on drawing an even, quiet stream of air in for a longer count.

Benefits: Balances the nervous system bringing the body into its natural (parasympathetic), restorative state. It is in this state where healing, digestion and nutrient absorption can take place.

Belly Breathing

Beginner

Exercise the lower lungs and release stored trauma and nervous tension in the solar plexus.

The Practice: Do this practice on an empty stomach. Sit tall and comfortably in a chair or lie flat on your back. Relax your belly fully and rest your hands there. Breathe in and out through your nose, with a steady, smooth, quiet breath, letting the belly rise and fall as you breathe. When developing this practice, actively push your belly out on the inhale (a sense of relaxing at your abdominal muscles) and actively draw your belly in on the exhale. As you develop this technique, the in and out motion of the belly becomes more subtle.

Benefits: Calms the mind; reduces anxiety (especially in the pit of the stomach); exercises the lower lungs; calms the nervous system; mitigates stress; reduces cravings; elevates serotonin and other feel good chemicals; improves the quality of sleep; improves memory and concentration.

Note: Many people unconsciously constrict their stomach, "sucking in" and creating unnecessary tension in the body. Belly breathing provides awareness of this tendency. Some discomfort may arise as you relax your core and let your belly come into its true form. Be mindful (compassionately self-aware) of any discomfort and tendency to constrict your core. Where else are you constricting, or holding on tightly in your life? Do you experience relief when you let your belly go?

-12-

Full Yogic Breathing

Intermediate (first practice the Belly Breathing)

Use this tool to optimize the breathing process, strengthen and heal the respiratory organs, and calm the nervous system (especially when experiencing high stress or anger).

Full yogic breathing differs from belly breathing in that it is a more expansive breath. Both the lower lungs and the upper lungs are filled and then emptied of breath.

The Practice: Start with belly breathing. When you're first starting out, rest one hand on your naval and one hand on the center of your chest (your heart). You may lie on your back or sit comfortably. Breathe smoothly and quietly in through your nose, first drawing the breath into the belly and letting it rise. Then continue your inhale until the chest too expands, filling the upper lungs. Pause at the top of your inhale, when both your lower and upper lungs are filled with breath. Then begin to control your exhale out through your nose, first letting air out of the upper lungs (chest will fall) and then drawing the belly gently in to encourage the breath out of the lower lungs. Pause at the bottom of your exhale. Continue to repeat this process with awareness on the quality of your breath—smooth, quiet, even, rhythmic, and full—and any sensation that arises. Do you feel a sense of calm wash over your body and mind?

Benefits: Strengthens the respiratory organs and softens the thoracic cavity; corrects and deepens natural breathing; maximizes the inhale and the exhale to increase oxygen intake and dispel stale carbon dioxide; purifies the blood; develops breath control; balances the nervous system.

-13-

Alternate Nostril Breathing

Intermediate (first practice Breath Control)

Balances masculine and feminine (sun and moon)
energies in the body for a more even, controlled
demeanor.

The Practice: This technique requires that you close off one nostril at a time. To do so, you'll use your ring finger and thumb, folding the pointer and middle fingers down. Begin by exhaling through your nose onto the back of one hand to identify which side is more congested (the nostril with the lighter stream of air). You will start by gently pressing the nostril with the lighter stream of air with the corresponding finger (ring finger or thumb). Ensure you're sitting tall with the eyes closed. With the proper nostril closed, gently draw your breath in through the open nostril for 3 to 5 seconds, then close that nostril, releasing and gently exhaling through the alternate nostril for the same length of time (3 to 5 seconds).

Tip: As you perfect this practice, focus on lengthening the in and out breaths and creating a quiet, eventually silent, smooth breath. You can tell your breath is smooth if you feel an even, soft stream of air against the inside of your nostrils on both the inhale and exhale. If one nostril feels especially closed, making this technique difficult or uncomfortable (indicative of an energy imbalance) it is time to use your Neti Pot!

Benefits: Balances hemispheres of the brain by balancing energy channels in the body (nadis); clears minor blockages in the nasal passage for even breathing through both nostrils.

-14-

Skull Shining Breath

(Kapalbhati Breathing)

Advanced

Cleansing for the lungs and energizing for mind.

Important! Do not practice if you are pregnant or have high blood pressure.

The Practice: As you practice this technique, your full awareness is on the exhale. The Skull Shining Breath involves a forceful exhale through the nose, with a passive inhale (the inhale happens automatically due to Pressure Differential). Sitting tall, gently place your hands on your belly. Start by bringing your awareness to your breath and taking a long, smooth breath in and out through your nose. Next take a short, smooth inhale and begin a series of 10 short, forceful exhales out through your nose. As the breath goes out, the belly will draw in (this is why it is helpful to have the hands there for awareness). Start with 3 sets of 10 exhales each, pausing between sets, remaining present for physical sensations and thoughts, and then initiating the next set of exhalations with a short, smooth inhale. As you develop this practice, increase to 20 breaths, 30, then 50 per set.

Benefits: Cleanses and strengthens the lungs; tones the digestive and abdominal organs; energizes the brain; clears water from the nasal passage after using your neti pot (see next page).

For neti pot instruction and benefits, see Practice 4, page 30 and 31.

Techniques for Performing Kapalbhati (Skull Shining) Breathing Post-Neti Pot:

Technique 1: From standing, bend over with your hands rested on your knees. Use Kapalbhati to expel water from your nostrils. Repeat for at least 2 sets of 10 breaths each.

Technique 2: Stand upright and jump up and down, with

the same forceful exhale through the nose. Jump up and push the breath/water out simultaneously 10 to 20 times.

Technique 3: Come into Downward Facing Dog Pose and use the same forceful breath. Take 10 exhalations looking to the left, 10 to the right, 10 looking at the naval, and 10 looking between your arms. Next come into Child's Pose for a few breaths. Repeat this process until the nasal passage feels clear and dry.

Note: It may take 10-20 minutes to clear all of the water from your nose. It is recommended to use a combination of the techniques above, pausing between repetitions and techniques.

Meditation Practices

"The gift of learning to meditate is the greatest gift you can give yourself in a lifetime."
–Sogyal Rinpoche

Meditation is therapy. For the purposes of this book, meditation can be defined as single-pointed focus on something other than your thoughts—such as the breath—while maintaining conscious awareness of your thoughts (rather than trying to stop them). Anyone can meditate, and there is no such thing as a good or bad meditator.

Consider the Buddhist analogy: thoughts are like clouds in the sky—unwavering, often out of our control, at times dark, thick, and stormy, at times light and fluffy, at times sparse, at times moving quickly, and at times slowly passing. As you meditate, watch your thoughts float by like clouds—intentionally choosing to disengage and let go for the time being (if it's important, it will come back)—and continuously return to your focal point.

It is important to note that you may have breakthroughs, epiphanies, or simply remember something you need to add to your "to do" list. This is an added benefit of meditation, but not the purpose of meditation. Regardless of what arises during, or the outcome of your practice, there is no end-goal of meditation and we do our best to fluidly move back into our day post-practice.

Meditation should be practiced regardless of your emotional and mental state; however, if you are in a depressive state, a dynamic or involved practice such as walking or flame meditation (page 76 to 79)—with the eyes open—or a guided meditation—recorded or in a group setting—may serve you more than a passive or silent practice.

Meditation allows space for mental clarity. In time, it teaches us that we can choose which thoughts we would like to give energy to; which thoughts we want to associate and identify with; and which we do not want to engage with, and therefore let float by. When practiced daily with compassionate self-awareness, we start to understand ourselves more fully—our triggers, our tendencies, our boundaries, our fears, our beliefs, our weakness', and our strengths become more apparent. Meditation gives us the opportunity to sift through the clutter of our mind and tune into our truth.

As we filter through thought patterns, limiting beliefs, and the stories we choose to represent ourselves with, we begin to see our true nature more clearly and realize our full potential. We can never clear away the clutter completely, but we can manage it with daily practice. If we miss a day, a week, a year, or ten years, we get right back to it.

Affirmation
I am not my thoughts and fears. I create my identity.

Fight-or-Flight

Daily meditation can change the brain. The average person has over 70,000 thoughts per day. The brain and nervous system do not differentiate between thoughts and our sensory experiences; thus, anxious, fear-based, or scarcity-driven thoughts can send the body into fight-or-flight the same way an external stimulus can (such as a house fire). In this inflammatory stress-state, the body mobilizes energy to prepare for survival; thus, natural bodily functions like digestion, nutrient absorption, and healing are not prioritized. Existing in this state during times of extreme danger is essential for rapid action and survival; however, existing in this state often is a recipe for poor health, undernourishment, exhaustion, and disease.

In time, with daily meditation practice, we train our brain to intercept this stress response. As our brain changes through meditation, we are able to access our rational thinking (neocortex) more quickly. We develop the awareness to breathe deeply through the nose and de-activate fight-or-flight in order to cultivate ease and acceptance in light of whatever may come our way.

* * * * *

Studying the benefits and theory behind meditation is less important than practicing and experiencing first hand how daily practice can transform you. Some of the common benefits of meditation include, but are not limited to: mental clarity, stress reduction, reduced rate of aging, self-realization, improved sleep, and better relationships. Use the following practices to incorporate meditation into your daily life: What do you learn about yourself?

66

Notes

What have you learned about yourself—your thinking, your body, your behaviors, your limiting beliefs—thus far?

-15-

Body Awareness Meditation

Learn to value your body as much as you value your mind; your feelings as much as your thinking.

Body awareness meditation is an excellent tool for learning to value your feelings just as much as you value your thinking (see page 42).

The Practice: Sit comfortably or lie down and simply tune in to your body. Notice what sensations you feel. Where do you feel tight or tense? What differences do you notice between the two sides of your body? Are you feeling energized or tired? Do you feel at peace or knots in your stomach? Notice when your thoughts chime in, and gently bring yourself back to your body (feelings and sensations).

Benefits: Develops mind-body connection; ripens the skill of thought-awareness; focuses the mind; establishes awareness and respect for the body.

Tip: Use this technique throughout your daily life. Recognize how you feel in your physical body. Do you feel energized and confident, only to feel the opposite when you look in the mirror, cannot find an outfit that you like, or receive constructive criticism from a colleague? Make an effort to notice when thoughts come in to prescribe negative judgment. How do your thoughts influence how you're feeling and visa versa? Thinking is powerful and can take us from feeling empowered to feeling small and uncomfortable in our own skin. Notice when this happens and recognize that you have not changed, only your thinking has changed.

-16-

Breath Awareness Meditation

Tune in to the four phases of your breath.

For anyone first starting out with meditation, this is a great technique to focus the mind and develop concentration.

The Practice: Focus on all four parts of your breath: the inhale, the space between the inhale and the exhale, the exhale, and the space between the exhale and the inhale. Pause and find stillness in the place where you are empty of breath (between the exhale and the inhale). Please note, this practice is different than breath control, as you are not intentionally altering the breath, you are simply watching it.

Tip: Let the in breath represent creation. With each inhale we are creating a new moment, and with a conscious inhale we have the ability to consciously create a positive thought or intention (see Practice 34, page 122 and 123). When we are conscious, we have the ability to make any moment exactly what we want it to be.

Let the exhale represent letting go. With each conscious exhale, we have the ability to consciously let something go: a thought, idea, story, sabotaging belief, tension in the body. Even if we just let go for a single moment, the more we practice letting go of something, the more likely we are to be able to let it go forever.

-17-

Sensory Awareness Meditation

Tune into each of your senses to seamlessly bring yourself into the present moment.

The Practice: Close your eyes and start by taking three full intentional breaths. Next, focus on each of your five of your senses, one at a time: What do you feel? What do you hear? What do you smell? What do you see behind your eyelids? What do you taste? Take 1-2 minutes to focus on each sensory experience you are having.

With awareness on each of your senses for about a minute or so, notice not only the obvious sensations, but search for layers of sensation: the quiet sounds in the background, the delicate textures and wisps of hair against your skin, your tongue against the roof of your mouth, the subtle tastes that linger on your palate.

Do this practice on its own, or use it to center and let go of distraction prior to another practice, such as Breath Awareness (see Practice 15, page 70 and 71) or affirming your goals (see Practice 37, page 128 and 129).

-18-

Walking Meditation and Earthing

Dynamic, grounding, and therapeutic.

Walking meditation is a dynamic practice, excellent for a group setting and for those needing to avoid introversion (especially people experiencing depression). The eyes are open and awareness is on physical sensation and what you see.

The Practice: Simply walk with your gaze down (if you prefer, you can lift your gaze and consciously observe your surroundings as you walk). Step with intention and notice the sensation that arises. Apply and refine your skill of compassionate awareness, aware of the tendency for your mind to drift away from the experience, or to judge the experience. If you are in a group, everyone can form and walk in a circle.

Earthing/Benefits: This practice is best done barefoot and outside on the grass, granite, or sand. As you connect your bare skin to the surface of the earth—whether walking, lying down, or practicing yoga— you absorb the planet's vast healing potential (free electrons), neutralizing inflammatory positive charges (pain and swelling)[1] in the body, and connecting to your original source. If you are in a scarcity mindset (see page 9) and are not feeling grounded, use this practice to connect with ground beneath you, feel supported, and cultivate gratitude for the earth.

For more information on the theory of Earthing, go to: www.earthinginstitute.net

-19-

Flame Meditation

Builds focus, exercises the eyes, calming before bed.

Also less of an introversive practice, flame meditation is mostly done with the eyes open.

The Practice: In a dark room, light a candle and simply watch the flame. Focus on one part of the flame at a time: the wick, the center, the tip, the aura around the flame. Stare intently at the flame for as long as you can without blinking. It is normal for the eyes to tear up and ache a little as you exercise them. Close the eyes for 5 to 10 seconds and repeat this process continuously for 5 minutes. As you get more experienced and make more time in your evening routine for self-care, extend this practice for 10 to 20 minutes.

Tip: Allow this practice to lead you into a long, resting posture (such as lying on your back), or guide you to sleep.

Benefits: Calming before bed; builds mental focus and concentration; exercises and strengthens the eye muscles.

-20-

Single-Pointed Focus

Focus the mind in one direction.

By now, you probably get the theme of meditation: single-pointed focus, or resting your awareness on one thing. The practices thus far have been more dynamic in nature, with various phases and focal points. As you hone in on the skill of focusing your mind, you can integrate a more passive practice into your repertoire.

The Practice: With eyes closed, rest your awareness on a single thing: your natural breath (without changing it), a soft, consistent noise, a soothing mental image (forest, waterfall, your favorite flower or landscape), your third eye (which rests inside, behind the space between your eyebrows), or a mantra (a sound you repeat silently to yourself).

An example of a mantra is "Om". You can repeat Om out loud, eventually getting quieter and quieter until the sound just resides in your head.

*　　*　　*　　*　　*

The skill of mindfulness can take years to develop and needs constant reinforcement. Daily meditation is the cement that keeps your foundation of compassionate awareness from crumbling. As you refine the practices in this chapter, mindfulness will naturally begin to penetrate your decisions, interactions, and relationships, enhancing your quality of life and deepening your sense of self. The eating practices that follow will further heighten your sense of self by providing your body and mind the nourishment to thrive. We can learn a lot about ourselves from the way that we eat and the foods that we choose.

Chapter Four

Nourish Your Body and Mind

Affirmation
I am what I eat.

The food we eat literally becomes our cells, blood, tissues, brain, thoughts, and reality. Food is a reflection of not only how we feel, but who we are and how effective we can be, as expressed in the following quotations.

"Tell me what you eat, I'll tell you who you are."
–Anthelme Brillat-Savarin

"One cannot think well, love well, sleep well, if one has not dined well."
—Virginia Wolfe

"The subtle energy of your food becomes your mind."
–The Upanishads

Your body, brain and soul require attention. The

Standard American Diet (SAD, see next page)—calorie-dense and nutrient-poor—is making people sick and sluggish. Consuming elements of the SAD on a regular basis makes achieving a healthy, abundant, and purposeful life more challenging because it depletes our vitality and clogs the body and thinking with toxic residue (see Chapter Two, page 19 to 22).

To support the process of implimenting long-term changes to the way you eat, it is important to paint your picture of wellness; to get clear on the standard of health that is important to you. Use Self-Awareness Exercise 2 (page 87) to clarify what health looks and feels like to you. Use your answers to come up with your own affirmations to support you in developing the belief that you can and will achieve your version of optimal health.

As you integrate the following eating habits into your daily life, you will have less space for the foods and habits that do not support your total well-being. Notice how you feel as you put nourishing food into your body whilst at the same time becoming more mindful of your eating process in general.

Standard American Diet (SAD)*

- High in processed or pulverized grains (flour products)
- High in sugar (soda, fruit juice, cane sugar, high fructose corn syrup—there are around 60 more different names for sugar in our food supply.)
- High in processed oils
- High in meat and animal fats
- Low in fresh fruits and vegetables (the RDV for fruits and vegetables is 7-10 servings, are you getting this? If not, you're likely to experience low energy and trouble concentrating, which leads to the next bullet point.)
- High in caffeine
- Low in whole grains (see page 96 and 97)
- Low in antioxidant-rich foods (see page 104 and 105)
- Low in Micro flora (probiotics, or beneficial bacteria, see page 106 and 107)
- Low in fiber

*If even one of these bullet points describes your *daily* diet, it is time to start making some serious changes so that you can show up energetically and for success.

*   *   *   *   *

True health is about a feeling. When we feel energized, confident, and in control, we can access health, abundance, and purpose with little effort. We can use food and the eating process to create natural energy in the body and give our cells the nutrients they need to thrive. With a healthy, whole foods diet, your entire demeanor and being will change. You will feel and appear more vital, the nature of your thoughts will improve, and you will wake up excited and intrigued for what is to come each day.

Follow these simple daily eating practices and you'll be well on your way toward achieving your healthiest self!

"Let food be thy medicine" *[not thy poison]*.
    -Hippocrates

Self-Awareness Exercise 2.

Imagine you are your healthiest in mind and body. Write down your answers to the questions below from the perspective of your healthiest self.

How do you feel when you wake up each morning and go to sleep at night?

What are your values and priorities?

What is your energy like?

What are the nature of your thoughts?

What are your accomplishments and goals?

Who do you surround yourself with?

How do you take care of yourself?

What foods do you eat?

What foods don't you eat?

Do you have a spiritual practice?

What do you do every single day?

How do you spend your free time?

What is the health of your family/children like?

Do you feel confident and in control of your life?

Notes

What does optimal health feel and look like to you? (Paint your picture of wellness.)

Notes

-21-

Drink Warm Lemon Water

A great pre-coffee morning ritual (or coffee replacement) to support digestion, detoxification, healthy aging, and immunity.

Drinking a glass of warm water with the juice of ¼ to ½ of a lemon in the morning or during the day can boost your Vitamin C and digestion.

A single lemon contains half of your body's recommended daily value of Vitamin C, a water-soluble antioxidant (needs to be continually replenished) that protects the body against free radical damage—characteristic of the aging process and the development of disease. Vitamin C is also critical for the production of glutathione (an important antioxidant for detoxification).

Lemon is antibacterial, astringent, and high in flavonoids to provide immunity against cold, flu, and bacterial and viral infections. It is also a digestive tonic, promoting peristaltic activity of the bowel and supporting healthy digestion and daily detox.

Although naturally acidic, lemon is actually alkalizing once it enters your body. Because much of the SAD (page 85) is acid-forming, this means that a daily dose of lemon water can support the body in maintaining its natural alkaline state.[2]

Tip: Steep ginger root in hot water, let cool until warm, then add lemon juice, a touch of cayenne pepper and raw honey for a tasty, awakening, digestive tonic! Rather than buying whole lemons (you'll go through a half per day), you can use a splash of store-bought organic lemon juice.

-22-

Do Not Drink Heavily With Meals

Chew, taste, and swallow your food instead of washing it down.

Drink a tall glass of room temperature water about 20 minutes prior to eating and again 20 minutes after eating for healthy digestion.

This practice prepares the body for digestion by lubricating the digestive tract and stimulating the production of bile (an important component of the digestive process) without washing out digestive enzymes in the mouth.

Note: You may notice that when you anticipate eating your mouth starts to salivate. Your saliva contains digestive enzymes that help to break down food before entering the stomach. Drinking liquids heavily with meals washes down and removes these digestive enzymes in the mouth, in addition to washing down under-chewed food (see Practice 31, page 110 and 111). Any food that is not broken down properly in the mouth puts an unnecessary strain on the digestive system. An inefficient digestive process can leave us feeling sluggish, uncomfortable, and toxic.

-23-

Eat Greens

kale, bok choy, parsley, cilantro, dandelion greens, collard greens, lettuce, spinach, mixed greens, arugula, swiss chard, beet greens, mustard greens

It's simple; eat greens everyday. Vary the greens you purchase each week, and buy organic whenever possible. If you're not able to buy organic, make sure to wash your greens thoroughly with a white vinegar and water mixture.

Leafy greens, by far, offer the most bang for your buck when it comes to micronutrient value. They are densely packed with phytochemicals (plant nutrients) and low in calories. Adopting this daily ritual can reduce oxidative stress (cellular aging), increase circulation, support daily detox, and get you that much closer to adequate nutrition.

Tip: To increase your daily dose of greens, combine a handful or two of chopped greens in your blender with a serving of fresh or frozen fruit (½ a banana, ½ cup berries, pineapple, watermelon, splash of lemon juice) and some fresh water, then blend and drink. You can also include other ingredients to make this more filling and flavorful: ½ avocado; raw nut butters; almond, soy, or regular milk; seeds (chia, hemp, or flax). Experiment with different ingredients and do your best to vary the fruits, greens, nuts and seeds you use.

-24-

Choose Whole Grains More Than Flour Products

*brown rice, wild rice, quinoa, barley, buckwheat,
millet, amaranth, oats, teff*

There is so much confusion these days about what constitutes a whole grain. The key to distinguishing between a whole grain and a processed grain is in the wording.

What does the word "whole" imply? Whole literally means that the grain is still in tact with all of its components: the fibrous husk (bran), the micronutrient-rich core (germ), and the carbohydrate-rich center (endosperm).

A processed, or fragmented, grain, is a grain that has been broken up and often stripped of its most nutritious elements (the germ and the bran), leaving the carbohydrate—a great source of energy, but void of micronutrients and dietary fiber. Any flour product is an example of a processed grain. A diet heavy in flour products (especially white and wheat flour) leads to blood sugar imbalance, energy crashes, fat storage, an inability to lose weight, insulin resistance, type 2 diabetes, and obesity.

Tip: Stay away from flour products *most* of the time. When choosing what to eat, opt for whole grains whenever possible. This choice will support you in feeling more energized in the short term and support your body in achieving and maintaining its ideal weight. In the long run, you will significantly increase your chances of living a long, healthy life.

-25-

Eat Raw Food Everyday

Strive to make 50% of your daily diet, and 50% of your plate, raw. Use this as a reference when you're building meals.

Raw food in its whole form has not been exposed to high temperatures (as is characteristic of refined food and the refinement process). Raw foods contain enzymes and the full range of micronutrients to help support the digestive process and assimilation of nutrients into the cells. Eating foods in their raw state also results in less metabolic waste, or less toxic buildup in the cells, which is generally higher in response to processed and cooked foods. Some examples of raw foods are, greens; fresh vegetables; fresh fruits; raw nuts and nut butters; and sprouted grains, seeds, and beans.

Tip: To mitigate the inflammatory response to cooked food and ensure you are getting a nutrient-dense diet, try to eat about half of your meals raw. If you plan to cook your veggies (which I love to do, especially with greens), keep at least half of them raw. You can massage raw course greens like kale, chard, and collards with avocado, olive oil and a little sea salt, then serve your raw and cooked greens together.

For more information on the importance of eating raw foods, see the work of David Wolfe and check out the documentary, Food Matters.

-26-

Eat Sea Veggies

arame, wakame, kelp, dulse, kombu

To adequately absorb vitamins, proteins and fats, your body needs minerals. Most people do not get adequate minerals (and micronutrients in general) in their daily diet. Mineral deficiencies can prevent the absorption of essential vitamins, enzymes, fats and proteins, leading to further deficiencies and compromising the body's internal systems and structures (e.g., bone loss and osteoporosis).

Tip: To boost your mineral intake and support healthy digestion, steam sea vegetables like kelp and kombu with your whole grains and cook them with your beans. Make stocks with kombu, nori and kelp. Add soaked wakame and arame to your salads and whole grains or mix in dulse flakes with mashed sweet potato and/or avocado dips.

Note: Sprinkling a ¼ teaspoon of organic sea salt on your food is another great way to get more minerals into your diet.

Increase Omega 3s and Reduce Omega 6s

Reduce chronic inflammation and your risk of disease.

Inflammation in the body is regulated by two essential fatty acids: Omega-3s and Omega-6s. These two fatty acids compliment each other, having opposite effects. The body draws from Omega-6s to construct pro-inflammatory hormones that increase clotting, cell proliferation, and blood flow to an area for healing. The body draws from Omega-3's to produce anti-inflammatory hormones that reduce those functions.

Ideally, we would be consuming these two fatty acids in roughly equal amounts, as humans did long ago during Paleolithic times. However, as the American diet has changed, the consumption of Omega-6s has come to far exceed that of Omega-3s. The major culprits of this imbalance are soybean oil (found in many processed foods) and grain fed meat or animal products, including dairy, which can be high in Arachidonic Acid (an Omega-6).

Tip: Increase Omega-3s in your diet by eating fatty fish like salmon, tuna, mackerel, bluefish and sardines, as well as walnuts, hemp seeds, chia seeds, and flax seeds. Or supplement with a highly pure, pharmaceutical-grade fish oil (see Practice 30, page 108 and 109 for more information).

-28-

Eat More Antioxidants

*blueberries, watercress, tomatoes, strawberries,
blackberries, cranberries, spinach, sweet potatoes,
broccoli, endive, apricots, kale, mango, papaya,
asparagus, cantaloupe, carrots* [3]

Antioxidants help the body cope with oxidative stress by neutralizing free radicals. Free radicals are highly reactive, natural by-products of metabolism and energy production. They are produced by the body in response to exposure to environmental toxins, food, inflammation, radiation, carcinogens, sun exposure, etc.

Tip: Make your meals colorful! In nature, antioxidants are expressed as color. As a general rule of thumb, eat a wide array of colors and get a wide array of anti-inflammatory, cancer-fighting micronutrients that support the body in aging more gracefully.

For more on antioxidants and antioxidant-rich foods reference the Nutrition Almanac [3]

-29-

Eat Cultured Foods for Probiotics

sauerkraut, kimchi, kefir, yogurt with live cultures,
unpasteurized dairy, raw apple cider vinegar, miso

The digestive tract (gut) houses a bacterial ecosystem integral to digestion and immunity. In fact, about 85% of the body's immune system lies within the gut lining, hence the strong relationship between the food we eat and how we feel.

The gut needs a diverse array of micro flora to remain resilient, strong, and for optimal digestion and disease prevention. In today's world, it is next to impossible to maintain a healthy micro flora balance. When this ecosystem becomes imbalanced due to depletion of "good" bacteria (e.g., Lactobacillus, Bifidus) or overgrowth of "bad" bacteria (e.g., candida)—due to frequent exposure to antibiotics or antibacterial products and a diet high in sugar and processed foods—the digestive and immune systems become compromised. This not only influences day-to-day well being, but impedes key cellular processes like DNA replication, cell turnover, and nutrient assimilation and absorption necessary for disease prevention.

Tip: Incorporate an array of cultured foods into your diet (like the ones listed to the left). Remember, diversity means resiliency. Keep in mind that these foods are living and therefore should not be exposed to high heat (do not cook or heat past boiling—in the case of miso soup) or enzymes in your mouth (until you're ready to eat them— e.g., avoid eating out of the container).

Fill in the Gaps With Pharmaceutical-Grade Supplements

Many Americans are lacking in key vitamins and minerals, like Vitamin B-12, Vitamin D, iron, zinc, and Omega 3 Fatty Acids. [4] *

*Seek the guidance of an experienced health professional to find a comprehensive regimen and brand to suit your needs.

Supplementation is key to maintaining optimal nutrition. Even for those of us who are diligent about eating the recommended 7-10 servings of fruits and vegetables each day, it is next to impossible to get the full range of vitamins and minerals in the correct ratios that the body needs to thrive (not just survive).

Of course, humans have not always relied on supplementation, but the food supply has changed significantly. The companies that regulate the bulk of our food supply put more emphasis on quantity and appearance than our nutrition. Companies like Monsanto and Cargill have normalized farming practices that boost output in the short term, while striping the soil of essential vitamins and minerals, resulting in visually appealing produce with depleted nutrition (tricky!).

Tip: Choose wisely! Much of the controversy around supplementation stems from the fact that it is an under-regulated industry. Many food-grade supplements may be ineffective and even harmful, with contaminants like heavy metals and inaccurate labels. When choosing a brand, ensure that it is pharmaceutical-grade and engineered for optimal absorption (such as Shaklee brand nutritional supplements). Look for scientific, peer-reviewed studies that indicate the products are safe and effective.

-31-

Chew Your Food

Chew each bite 20 to 30 times (at least).

You are what you digest. Ensure you are getting optimal nutrition from your food and not over-taxing your digestive system (also see Practice 22, page 92 and 93).

Chewing is the most important part of the digestive process. When we are truly hungry and we anticipate eating—by smelling and seeing food—we salivate. Salivation is a sign that the digestive system is fired up; digestive juices are flowing and the body is prepared to process and assimilate the food we are about to eat. Within the saliva are digestive enzymes crucial to efficient digestion. The longer you chew and hold food in your mouth, exposing it to digestive enzymes and masticating it fully, the less work it takes for your body to break down the food down once it enters your stomach.

Tip: Next time you sit down to eat, set an intention to chew each bite at least 20 times (some recommend 30 and up to 50). Notice if your mouth starts to salivate as you anticipate eating, this means your digestive system is ready to work! As you eat, focus on chewing, tasting, absorbing nutrition, and digesting your food.

-32-

Eat Mindfully

Get more nourishment and pleasure from your food.

The way we eat is equally important as what we eat. When we are fully present for what and how we're eating, we can derive more *sustained* pleasure from the eating experience, and our tendency to overeat or eat foods that do not serve us is reduced. Additionally, if we are stressed, tense, anxious and unaware when we eat, the digestive process is compromised, resulting in low energy, digestive distress (IBS, diarrhea, constipation), and sub-optimal nutrition from our food—healthy or not (See Fight-or-Flight, page 67).

Mindful Eating Tips

1. Light a candle before you eat (and maybe even as you cook) to ritualize the experience and create a relaxed ambiance.

2. Reserve a moment before digging in to cherish your food and bring mindfulness into the eating process, whatever this means to you: 3 deep breaths, expressing gratitude to the chef (even if its you!), noticing the aromas of the food, imagining where the food came from, or saying grace or some other form of prayer.

3. As you chew thoroughly (see previous practice), bring your full awareness to the flavor profiles of the foods and the simple act of chewing. Try not to distract yourself from the chewing process by watching TV or reading. Of course, eating in loving company is the best way to eat, so in this situation, we multi-task.

4. Set your utensil down between bites, chewing and swallowing each bite fully before taking another. I like to use chopsticks when I can; this encourages me to take

smaller bites and forces me to slow down.

5. Continue to check in with your senses, your breath, and your body throughout the meal. Ask yourself: *Am I satisfied?* Stop when you are! Be mindful of what thoughts and feelings arise as you eat and after you're done: are they negative or positive? What eating behaviors lead to which thoughts?

The most important part of mindful eating is to thoroughly enjoy your food; both for the taste and life-giving nutrients it is providing you.

Chapter Five

Self-Realize and Get What You Want

Affirmation

Thank you so much for aligning my dreams and affirmations with my reality.

Now that you have the tools to establish and maintain a strong foundation of health, it is time to connect with your true nature, articulate your life purpose, and realize your full potential—all of which are determined by your beliefs and values. The practices that follow are here to help you get clear on what you believe, what you want to create, and how you want to influence the world around you.

I have recently been inspired by the work of Dan Beuttner and his research on Blue Zones[5], or longevity hubs—small pockets throughout the world where most people remain healthy and disease-free as they age. According to the findings of Dan Beuttner and his team, people who not only feel a strong sense of purpose, but can state it in one sentence or less, live an average of eight years longer than those who cannot. This makes sense, as those who have a strong sense of purpose have a guiding light, a reason for being that motivates action, supports mental clarity, and fosters ease despite uncertainty.

Use Self Awareness Exercise 3 (see page 118) and the following practices to guide you toward identifying and living for your life's purpose. As your guiding light burns brighter, you can use this clarity to recognize how you can live your purpose wholeheartedly for a more fulfilled life. You can also determine circumstances, behaviors, thoughts, beliefs and relationships that dim the light and take the necessary action to make changes.

*   *   *   *   *

When we are clear on and act in alignment with our beliefs, purpose and values, we are less weighted down by resistance in the form of stress, anxiety, fear, jealousy, and judgment. As this resistance is lifted, we see clearly our true nature and do not feel so inhibited by the day-to-day tasks. Instead, we can find in almost any task an opportunity to represent our true selves and connect with our purpose. How do you want to show up in the world today? How do you want to show up for others? How do you want to influence the planet? What do you want to project?

When we are clear on our true nature—as reflected in our deepest beliefs about who we are—and act accordingly, we get more fulfillment from our actions, allowing us to exude a presence of peace, softness, ease, and acceptance. The practices in this section are here to help you lift the weight of resistance by getting clear on who you really are and what you want to create and

114

contribute to each day of your life. Remember, your belief creates your identity; you decide who you are. With daily practice, you can develop the clarity to manifest your deepest desires and realize your potential.

Self-Awareness Exercise 3.

Use your answers to the questions below to articulate your life's purpose.

What do you value?

What do you believe about yourself? (What kind of person are you?)

What are your strengths?

What brings you lasting pleasure?

What causes you regret, stress or anxiety?

What do you resist or dislike doing?

When do you feel most present and at peace? (Is there a behavior that triggers this?)

Still not sure?

What gets you out of bed each day? What do you want to share with the world, or learn from the world? What, within yourself, do you want to stay true to every single day? What brings you peace despite the underlying uncertainty of our existence?

Your purpose can be simple, such as:

To inspire others to love unconditionally.

To be a source of joy and laughter for others.

To practice and teach mindfulness.

Keep in mind, your purpose may evolve as you do.

My Values:

My Personal Beliefs:

My Strengths:

What I want to share with the world is...

My life purpose is...

-33-

Ask Why?

Know your why.

Why are you reading this book? Why do you do anything you do? These questions may seem silly, but when articulated, the answers can be quite powerful. Equally as powerful can be your lack of reasoning.

When we take the time to reflect on *why*, we can consciously identify if a behavior is aligned with our beliefs, values, and purpose. If we take this a step further and let our reflection drive our daily decisions, our behaviors and choices become more intentional and we feel closer to our true selves.

The Practice: Identify one thing you do each day and journal about why you do it. Examples include: drinking coffee, going to work, taking a yoga class, or meditating. As you consider why, also reflect on how your actions, purchases, relationships, and behaviors enrich or exhaust your joy and that of those around you.

Tip: Utilize this process with respect to any/all of your tasks, relationships, investments (temporal and monetary), and behaviors. Overtime, this awareness of *why* will guide your decisions about who you interact with and where you direct your energy. This is also a great tool to bring yourself back to your purpose when feeling lost in the day-to-day grind. Throughout this process remember to be mindful: Have compassion for yourself and your experiences.

-34-

Be Intentional

(And put it in ink.)

Asking why and developing intentions are closely linked. When we ask why, our behaviors and decisions become more intentional.

The Practice: Take time in the morning to set one or more intentions for the day ahead. Ask yourself: *What do I want to work on today? What do I want to radiate? What do I need more of in my life? What do I need less of?* Write it down.

Tip: Your intention is different than a goal or item on your "to-do" list (although putting it on there may be effective). Let your intention be something you can practice in each moment, a trait or feeling that you can embody right now, rather than some future oriented goal. Future goals are excellent tools for personal growth, but they are different than intentions. An example of a future goal would be: *To get the job I am interviewing for today.* Rather, your intention could be: *Exude confidence and professionalism.*

More examples of intentions include: *"be present", "practice non-judgment", "accept myself", "radiate positivity", "do my best", "be a better listener", "ask more questions", "enjoy", "let go"…*

-35-

Three Gratitudes

Nurture the mindset of abundance and connect with a force larger than yourself.

Gratitude helps us remain humble. When we express our gratitude to something bigger than ourselves (I often use the Universe, some may use God), we nurture the belief that we, as well as our achievements and contributions, are vehicles of a greater connective force that drives all of existence. Expressing gratitude for the pieces of our existence that bring us joy and ascribing these phenomena to a source both within and greater than ourselves reminds us each day that our life is an incredible gift, one to be maximized and not taken lightly.

The Practice: Take time at the end of each day to write down three things that you appreciate, are thankful for, or that went well that day. Ask yourself, *what's going well in my life?* Be specific. After you write down your gratitudes, close your eyes and express thanks to the greater connective force that ultimately makes all of this possible.

Tip: This practice is especially powerful during difficult or challenging times. Noticing glimpses of positivity can pull us out of the scarcity mindset and into a mindset of abundance (see page 10).

-36-

Know and Affirm Who You Are and What You Want

You decide who you are, and who you are decides your future.

Becoming clear on what we want is the first step toward achieving it. The second step is cultivating belief that you can (see Self-Awareness Exercise 1, page 16). As you know, affirmations (see definition, page 7) help us identify, articulate, and believe in what we will create and who we are.

The Practice: Think of a time when you have undervalued yourself, or identified with a way of being that made you feel small: for example, *I am indecisive* or *I am weak*. Each time we make such statements, whether spoken in our mind or out loud, it is an affirmation, a declaration of something that you are. Recognize the power of *I am* and shift your statements to reflect the person you want to be. For example, *I am strong, I am decisive, I make decisions quickly and without regret*.

Tip: Create a Vision Board that conveys what you want to accomplish this year or in your lifetime. Use pictures cut out from magazines and language that you find or write yourself to exemplify what you want and who you are. Post your vision board somewhere visible as a daily reminder of what you are creating. Ensure to tune into your vision daily, aligning your energy and awareness with what you are working toward.

-37-

Set Clear Goals and Action Steps

"Great visions precede great achievements."
-John Maxwell

Goals and action steps are integral components of self-realization, essential for forward thinking and action; they are the nuts and bolts necessary to realize our potential.

The Practice: Break down your long-term goals into short-term goals and daily action steps. Start an on-going list of life goals. Be aware of and begin to address limiting beliefs as they arise (see page 10). Next, develop a list of goals for the year to come. Where do you envision yourself one year from today? At the start of each month, write down your goals for the month ahead. What do you want to accomplish to take you closer to your yearly and lifetime goals? On Sunday evening or Monday morning, write down your goals for the week ahead. Lastly, reserve 5-minutes each morning to write down action steps that will guide you closer to your weekly, monthly, yearly, and life goals.

Tip: Post your goals somewhere obvious and look at them every day, checking them off and adapting them as necessary. We all know that life does not always go as planned, in which case we need to be willing to compassionately readjust our goals and action steps in order to stay action oriented.

Turn your goals into affirmations by bringing them into the present tense. For example, if your goal is to de-clutter your living space, your affirmation could be: *I am clutter free.*

-38-

Take Daily Action

*"Vision without action is merely a dream.
Action without vision just passes the time.
Vision with Action can change the world."*
-Joel A. Barker

Aside from stating your goals and affirmations, there are three essential components to realizing what you want:

1. The belief in yourself (see Self-Awareness Exercise 1, page 16).

2. Knowing why (see Practice 33, page 120 and 121).

3. Taking action.

The Practice: Do at least one thing every day to whittle away at your goals. Your daily action may be tangible, such as scheduling a meeting with your boss to discuss your future, or more abstract, such as reading a book to enhance your knowledge or shift your thinking. When feeling overwhelmed with all life is throwing at you, slow down, breathe, ground yourself in your why and purpose, and ask yourself: *What can I do right now?*

Note: Acknowledge your action, despite the outcome. When we take action there is always the potential for failure. Learn from challenges and failures, but use your underlying belief in yourself, long-term vision, and sense of purpose to access the motivation to move forward regardless of the outcome; failure is just one stop along the road to success!

-39-

Evaluate and Reduce Your Impact

What footprint do you want to leave on the planet?

As we gain more control and abundance in our life through daily practice, we develop the wherewithal to make decisions in favor of the greater social and planetary good. Start to evaluate the hidden environmental and human costs of your day-to-day actions. The food you buy, the clothes you wear, the amount of packaging on these products, the waste you produce. How can you reduce the hidden impacts of your actions?

The Practice: Educate yourself on the major industries you interact with and how they influence not only planetary health, but human health as well. I recommend watching the following documentaries. Let what you learn guide your daily decision-making.

Food Inc, the costs of food production in America.

The True Cost, the underlying costs of the global fashion industry.

Inhabit, permaculture as a way to live in accordance with the laws of nature and stimulate regeneration of agricultural, eco- and, economic systems.

An Inconvenient Truth, one of the most important films of our time to inspire sustainable action against climate change.

A Few Tips to Reduce Your Impact

Buy Organic: Not just food, choose clothes produced with organic cotton. In general, these products are less supportive of practices that harm human and environmental health, and in doing so you'll reduce your exposure to toxic residue that persists on non-organic clothing.

Reduce Your Waste: Stop buying paper towels. You'll be surprised by how easy life is without them. Pretty soon, you'll get used to using a dish towel or cloth napkin, just like our grandparents did before the age of convenience.

Detoxify Your Home: Buy non-toxic, concentrated cleaners. The average household cleaner is made up of chemical concentrate mixed with mostly water. The inefficiency and environmental impact of shipping water and packaging across the country is sickening. Even more striking, have you ever read the label on your household cleaner?

Cleaners are among the most toxic substances found in homes and contribute to indoor air pollution, causing respiratory distress, allergies, poisonings, and asthma (especially among children).[4] Replace toxic cleaners and detergents with non-toxic concentrate (we've all heard the vinegar and water trick), such as Shaklee brand cleaners, which require that you add your own water. Not only will this action reduce toxic residue in your home, but it will lighten your environmental footprint *and* save you money.

Integrating these practices will reduce the human and environmental destruction associated with the production and consumption of cheap, disposable consumer goods.

On a personal level, as we identify and commit to our values, we feel more trusting of ourselves, and we begin to hold ourselves to a higher standard of behavior. When we respect ourselves, this self-respect radiates outward and we continue to attract abundance.

-40-

Fuel Your Passion

Identify what ignites you and go do it!

What is most important to you? If this were your last day in the earth, how would you spend it? Think back to a time when you felt immense joy in your life: What was driving that? When do all of your worries drift away?

The Practice: Identify one daily, weekly, monthly, or yearly practice that nurtures your inner flame, such as: taking a walk in nature, volunteering in favor of the planet and greater good, writing, swimming in the ocean, climbing a mountain. If you haven't already, determine what fuels your passion and create a ritual around it.

Tip: Schedule a time each day, week, month, or year for your ritual. Notice if your mind starts to come up with stories or excuses as to why you do not have the time, but make an effort to stick to your schedule. *Do you feel differently when you are taking this time to fuel your passion, versus when you are prioritizing everything else?*

Conclusion

I hope your journey through this book has guided you to make a habit of caring for yourself. We live in a culture where everything else takes precedence to our own self-care. We are often taught to "put others before ourselves". While this selfless paradigm is noble in theory, is it sustainable? I think not.

The destruction of our planet and the chronically stressed and high cortisol state that many people exist in is in part a result of this very mindset. We put our work, families, even strangers before ourselves. And when we do take time for ourselves, we are so disconnected from what we are actually seeking—what brings us sustained enjoyment—that we spend our time distracting ourselves away from the voids and imbalances that we have created—we watch TV, overeat food that is making us sick, drink heavily, use drugs. And the worst part is, as we feed this cycle of poor health, lack of time, planetary destruction, unawareness, and disconnect, we are left hungry and seeking more.

The solution? Take time to connect with yourself everyday; with your needs, desires, goals, gratitudes, and dreams. Rather than just letting life happen to you, create the life you want by constantly reflecting on how you could feel better and be better. When we feel healthy, abundant, and purposeful, we show up stronger for others, and we are better able to support the planet on which we live. When we take care of ourselves, we are able to be present for our children, our partners, our friends, even complete strangers. By taking time to connect to ourselves, we connect more deeply to others and we make them feel heard.

Self-care is something you identify for yourself. Self-care is anything that brings more harmony, joy, and peace into your life. I hope that the rituals in this book guide you to better understand what daily practices support *your* health, inner fulfillment, and sense of purpose.

Be patient with yourself throughout this process of transformation. Have compassion and know that setbacks are normal. If and when you feel things spiraling out of control, take a step back, close your eyes, take three deep breaths, and ask yourself: *What can I do right now to reconnect to my purpose?*

The point of all of this is to get more sustained enjoyment out of life. To live with less dis-ease, angst, regret, and resentment. To be present for your life and achieve the very best version of yourself. To wake up!

Now, start practicing.

Glossary

Abundance Mindset: A learned tendency to notice the abundance of beauty and good in your life, with a willingness to take responsibility for and address dissatisfaction by making tangible changes or shifting your thinking.

Affirmation: An assertive, present-tense statement of something as fact. It is usually an *I am* or *I have* statement used to shift your thinking. Cultivating belief in that which you are affirming is the most important part of an affirmation practice.

Affirmative Belief: A belief that encourages a positive mental outlook and creates (rather than restricts) possibility and opportunity; thus, supports abundance and action.

Awareness: The ability to watch and observe your inner and outer landscape, as well as that of others, without judgment or the need to find answers/understand.

Judgment: The tendency to label an emotion, place, behavior, person, thought, circumstance, or the self favorably or unfavorably; a necessary component of decision-making and intentional action.

Limiting Belief: An acquired belief that holds you back from taking action; thus, limiting your potential.

Mindfulness: The ability to observe your present moment with compassion and awareness; compassionate self-awareness.

Scarcity Mindset: A tendency to perceive what is lacking in your life, often infused with negative judgment, blame, and an inability to take responsibility for your discontent.

Self-Awareness: Knowledge and awareness of your own personality, character, reactions, tendencies, thoughts, beliefs, values, and purpose; a skill that allows you to be the conscious observer of your thoughts and feelings and to take intentional action.

Self-Care: Any deliberate action taken by an individual to uphold and enhance their health and well being; an expression of self-love.

Yoga: A conscious process toward growth; a systematic methodology for well-rounded personality development—physical, mental, intellectual, emotional and spiritual. Yoga techniques—including, but not limited to, postures (asanas), breathing techniques (pranayama), and meditation—work on the body and the mind to establish even-mindedness and well being, bringing the individual into a state of control, stability and acceptance.

References and Suggested Reading

[1] *Earthing: The most important health discovery ever?* by Clinton Ober, Stephen Sintara, M.D. and Martin Zucker. Basic Health Publications, Inc., 2010

[2] *Encyclopedia of Natural Medicine, 3rd Edition,* by Michael T, Murray, ND and Joseph Pizzorno, MD. Atria, 2012.

[3] *Nutrition Almanac, 6th Edition* by John D. Kirschmann and Nutrition Search, Inc. McGraw Hill, 2007.

[4] *Why Do I Feel This Way? Understand Your Body...Discover You Solutions* by Christine Gaber, RHN and Charlne Day, RDC. Health Through Knowledge, 2012.

[5] *Blue Zones: Eating and Living Like the Worlds Healthiest People* by Dan Beuttner. National Geographic Society, 2015

Diet for a Small Planet by Frances Moroe Lappe. Ballantine Books, 1991

The Happiness Advantage by Shawn Achor. Crown Business, 2010

Integrative Nutrition: Feed your Hunger for Health and Happiness by Joshua Rosenthal. Integrative Nutrition, 2014

About the Author

Allie Andrews is deeply passionate about people, food, health, dance, yoga, and nurturing connection to the earth. Ever since she was seven years old, she knew she had to be connected to the outdoors. As a student of Environmental Science, Conservation Biology, and Permaculture, she spent her college years and the early portion of her adult life investigating the human influence on the natural world.

As Allie's thinking evolved, she began to see the problem as the solution: there is an immense disconnect from the self and the outcomes of our actions that must be cured in order to heal the planet. Allie's motivation shifted from protecting the environment and advocating for behavioral change on a large scale, to pursuing a career as a health coach and yoga teacher in order to guide people to love, respect, and take care of themselves.

Some of Allie's favorite and most formative life experiences include through-hiking the Appalachian Trail and studying yoga in India. Allie views life as an adventure in personal growth and transformation. She is dedicated to teaching and practicing mindfulness through her work and uses her expertise to elevate health in corporate cultures.

Connect with Allie

OmBodyHealth.com

allie@ombodyhealth.com

www.facebook.com/ombodyhealth

Instagram: @ombodyhealth

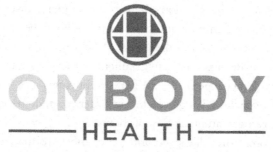

Made in United States
North Haven, CT
04 October 2021

10145228R00085